THE *Skinny*
NUTRiBULLET
LEAN BODY
HiiT PLAN

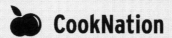 CookNation

THE SKINNY NUTRIBULLET LEAN BODY HIIT PLAN

DELICIOUS CALORIE COUNTED SMOOTHIES & JUICES WITH HIGH INTENSITY INTERVAL TRAINING WORKOUTS FOR A LEANER, FITTER YOU

ISBN 978-1-911219-35-4

A CIP catalogue record of this book is available from the British Library

• •

DISCLAIMER

This book is designed to provide information on smoothies and juices that can be made in the NUTRiBULLET appliance only, results may differ if alternative devices are used.

A basic level of fitness is required to perform the workouts in this book. Any health concerns should be discussed with a health professional before embarking on any of the exercises detailed.

The NutriBullet™ is a registered trademark of Homeland Housewares, LLC. Bell & Mackenzie Publishing is not affiliated with the owner of the trademark and is not an authorized distributor of the trademark owner's products or services.
This publication has not been prepared, approved, or licensed by NutriBullet ™ or Homeland Housewares, LLC.

Some recipes may contain nuts or traces of nuts. Those suffering from any allergies associated with nuts should avoid any recipes containing nuts or nut based oils.
This information is provided and sold with the knowledge that the publisher and author do not offer any legal or other professional advice.
In the case of a need for any such expertise consult with the appropriate professional.
This book does not contain all information available on the subject, and other sources of recipes are available.

This book has not been created to be specific to any individual's or NUTRiBULLET's requirements.
Every effort has been made to make this book as accurate as possible. However, there may be typographical and or content errors. Therefore, this book should serve only as a general guide and not as the ultimate source of subject information.

This book contains information that might be dated and is intended only to educate and entertain.

The author and publisher shall have no liability or responsibility to any person or entity regarding any loss or damage incurred, or alleged to have incurred, directly or indirectly, by the information contained in this book.

CONTENTS

NUTRIBLASTS UNDER 400 CALORIES

HIGH INTENSITY INTERVAL TRAINING WORKOUTS

OTHER COOKNATION TITLES

INTRODUCTION

Our smoothies & workouts will set you on a lifelong path to a healthier, leaner and happier you!

If you are reading this you will likely already have purchased a NUTRiBULLET or perhaps are considering buying one. A smart choice! The NUTRiBULLET is unquestionably one of the highest performing smoothie creators on the market. Its clean lines and compact design look great in any kitchen. It's simple to use, easy to clean and the results are amazing.

You may have watched or read some of the NUTRiBULLET marketing videos and literature which make claims of using the power of the NUTRiBULLET to help you lose weight, boost your immune system and fight a number of ailments and diseases. Of course the 'healing' power comes from the foods we use to make our smoothies but the real difference with the NUTRiBULLET is that it EXTRACTS all the goodness of the ingredients. Unlike many juicers and blenders, which leave behind valuable fibre, the NUTRiBULLET pulverises the food, breaking down their cell walls and unlocking the valuable nutrients so your body can absorb and use them.

You may have made your own smoothies in the past using a blender – you'll know even with a powerful device that there are often indigestible pieces of food left in your glass – not so with the NUTRiBULLET which uses 600 watts to breakdown every part of the food. The manufacturer calls it 'cyclonic action' running at 10,000 revolutions per minute but whatever the marketing jargon, the results speak for themselves.

The NUTRiBULLET is not a blender and not a juicer. It is a nutrient extractor, getting the very best from every ingredient you put in and delivering a nutrient packed smoothie called a 'Nutriblast'. Using the power of the NUTRiBULLET is an incredibly fast and efficient way of giving our bodies the goodness they need. Making the most of anti-oxidants to protect your cells, omega 3 fatty acids to help your joints, fibre to aid digestion and protein to build and repair muscles.

Just one nutrient packed Nutriblast a day can make a difference to the way you feel and it only takes seconds to make!

All our recipes make use of the tall cup of the NUTRiBULLET and the extractor blade. Feel free to experiment. Mixing your ingredients is fun and will help your create wonderful new combinations too. As a basic formula, work on 50% leafy greens 50% fruit, ¼ cup of seeds/nuts and water.

There has never been a better time to introduce health-boosting, weight reducing, well-being smoothies to your life. With a spiralling obesity epidemic in the western world which in turn is linked to a growing list of debilitating diseases and ailments including diabetes, high blood pressure, heart disease, high cholesterol, infertility, skin conditions and more, the future for many of us can look bleak. Combine this with the super-fast pace of modern life and we can be left feeling fatigued and lethargic, worsened by daily consumption of unhealthy foods.

The good news is that you have taken a positive step to improve your life. The power of the NUTRiBULLET, our delicious calorie counted smoothies and high intensity workouts are a killer combination and will set you on the path to a leaner, fitter body.

THE HIIT PLAN WORKOUTS

If you are new to regular exercise or haven't been active for some time then firstly congratulations on making a positive step to getting back into shape! Exercise is a great way to improve not just your body but also your mind. Not only can regular physical activity help prevent illness it can also bring clarity and focus to your everyday life. It can help you lose weight, get trim and keep you feeling better. There are many benefits to reap from regular exercise.

Before starting on our HiiT workouts it is important to evaluate your basic level of fitness. If you have any major health concerns such as those listed below we recommend first seeking a health professionals advice.

- Heart disease
- Asthma or lung disease
- Type 1 or type 2 diabetes
- Kidney disease
- Arthritis

- Pain or discomfort in your chest
- Back pain
- Dizziness or light-headedness
- Shortness of breath
- Ankle swelling

- Rapid heartbeat
- Smoker
- Overweight
- High blood pressure
- High Cholesterol

If you are or think you may be pregnant we do not recommend you undertake these workouts.

HiiT, or high-intensity interval training, is a new kind of training program which concentrates on you giving your maximum effort through fast, intense bursts of exercise, followed by short recovery periods. It is quick and convenient and does not require equipment so you can do it anywhere, anytime.

These predominantly cardio exercises are designed to get your heart rate up, which in turn burns more fat in less time by increasing the body's need for oxygen during the effort. This creates an oxygen shortage, causing your body to ask for more oxygen during recovery. Often referred to as Excess Post-Exercise Oxygen Consumption (EPOC) this is the reason why intense exercise helps burn more fat and calories than traditional aerobic/cardio workouts.

Put simply regular HiiT workouts will help you increase your metabolism, reduce body fat and build lean muscle. In order to do this effectively our HiiT workouts should be combined with a healthy nutritional lifestyle, which is why the calorie counted NUTRiBULLET recipes in this book are the perfect partner. You should however not rely solely on our recipes as your daily nutritional intake. Physical and indeed everyday activities require energy to perform so we recommend a balanced diet of carbohydrates, protein and fat. Using a fitness tracker such as MyFitnessPal will help you achieve your daily nutritional needs.

Prior to performing any physical activity make sure you warm up first with some gentle stretching and exercises such as jogging on the spot and jumping jacks (see workouts from page 76).

We have compiled 4 high intensity interval training workouts to perform each week (see page 73). To begin with ease yourself into these exercises especially if it has been some time since you have engaged in any cardio based training. As you progress and feel more comfortable with the routines you can increase intensity.

You should aim to do all 4 workouts within a 7 day period (1 per day) using the remaining 3 days to rest. Try to alternate where possible between training and rest days. Rest days are important as they give your body time to recover and repair - don't be tempted to skip them. Each workout lasts for approximately 15 minutes and a simple explanation with diagrams of how to correctly perform each exercise is provided.

Over time conditioning routines (HiiT) will help to make you lean in conjunction with a healthy balanced diet. They take work, time and dedication so be sure to stick at them and increase the intensity as the weeks go by. As you progress you can, if you wish, start to introduce some basic weights (such as light dumbbells) into some of the exercises such as squats, lunges and standing mountain climbers. Devoting just 15 mins of your day to keep fit will set you on a lifelong path to a healthier, leaner and happier you.

WORKOUT TIPS

- Remember to breathe through each exercise
- Have a bottle of water to drink from between sets
- Always warm up and cool down before and after each workout
- Keep your core tight and give maximum effort
- Enjoy!

NUTRIBULLET TIPS

To help make your Nutriblast fuss-free, follow these quick tips.

- Prepare your shopping list. Take some time to select which Nutriblasts you want to prepare in advance. As with all food shopping, make a note of all the ingredients and quantities you need. Depending on the ingredients it's best not to shop too far in advance to ensure you are getting the freshest produce available. We recommend buying organic produce whenever you can if your budget allows. Organic produce can give a better yield and flavour to your Nutriblast. Remember almost all fruit is fine to freeze too.
- Cut up any produce that may not fit into the tall cup, but only do this just before making your smoothie to keep it as fresh as possible.
- Wash your Nutriblast parts immediately after juicing. As tempting as it may be to leave it till a little later you'll be glad you took the few minutes to rinse and wash before any residue has hardened.
- Substitute where you need to. If you can't source a particular ingredient, try another instead. More often than not you will find the use of a different fruit or veg makes a really interesting and delicious alternative. In our recipes we offer some advice on alternatives but have the confidence to make your own too!
- To save time prepare produce the night before for early morning Nutriblasts.

- Wash your fruit and veg before juicing. This needn't take up much time but all produce should be washed clean of any traces of bacteria, pesticides and insects.
- Some Nutriblasts are sweeter than others and it's a fact that some of the leafy green drinks can take a little getting used to. Try drinking these with a straw, you'll find them easier to drink and enjoy.

IMPORTANT — WHAT NOT TO USE IN YOUR NUTRIBLASTS

The manufacturers of NUTRiBULLET are very clear on the following warning. While the joy of making Nutriblasts is using whole fruit and vegetables there are a few seeds and pits which should be removed. The following contain chemicals which can release cyanide into the body when ingested so do not use any of the following in your Nutriblasts:

- Apple Seeds
- Cherry Pits
- Peach pits
- Apricot Pits
- Plum Pits

CLEANING

Cleaning the NUTRiBULLET is thankfully very easy. The manufacturer gives clear guidelines on how best to do this but here's a recap:

- Make sure the NUTRiBULLET is unplugged before disassembling or cleaning.
- Set aside the power base and blade holders as these should not be used in a dishwasher.
- Use hot soapy water to clean the blades but do not immerse in boiling water as this can warp the plastic.
- Use a damp cloth to clean the power base.
- All cups and lids can be placed in a dishwasher.
- For stubborn marks inside the cup, fill the cup 2/3 full of warm soapy water and screw on the milling blade. Attach to the power base and run for 20-30 seconds.

WARNING:

Do not put your hands or any utensils near the moving blade. Always ensure the NUTRiBULLET is unplugged when assembling/disassembling or cleaning.

ABOUT CookNation

CookNation is the leading publisher of innovative and practical recipe books for the modern, health conscious cook. CookNation titles bring together delicious, easy and practical recipes with their unique approach - easy and delicious, no-nonsense recipes - making cooking for diets and healthy eating fast, simple and fun.

With a range of #1 best-selling titles - from the innovative 'Skinny' calorie-counted series, to the 5:2 Diet Recipes collection - CookNation recipe books prove that 'Diet' can still mean 'Delicious'!

THE *Skinny*
NUTRiBULLET
LEAN BODY
HiiT PLAN

NUTRIBLASTS UNDER 200 CALORIES

CARROT, APPLE & RASPBERRY JUICE

190 calories

Ingredients

- 75g/3oz raspberries
- 1 apple
- 125g/4oz carrots
- Water

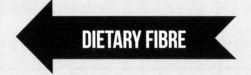

DIETARY FIBRE

Method

1 Rinse the ingredients well.

2 Core the apple. Top & tail the carrots, no need to peel.

3 Add the raspberries & carrots to the NUTRiBULLET tall cup. Make sure the ingredients do not go past the MAX line on your machine.

4 Add water, again being careful not to exceed the MAX line.

5 Twist on the NUTRiBULLET blade and blend until smooth.

CHEF'S NOTE

Carrots contain beta-carotene which the body converts to Vitamin A.

STRAWBERRY COCONUT MILK SMOOTHIE

198 calories

Ingredients

- 25g/1oz spinach
- 75g/3oz strawberries
- 120ml/½ cup low fat coconut milk
- 1 tsp honey
- Water

Method

1 Rinse well and remove the green tops from the strawberries.

2 Add the honey, spinach strawberries & coconut milk to the NUTRiBULLET tall cup. Make sure the ingredients do not go past the MAX line on your machine.

3 Add a little water if needed to take it up to the MAX line.

4 Twist on the NUTRiBULLET blade and blend until smooth.

CHEF'S NOTE

This is a naturally sweet & light smoothie. Serve with lots of crushed ice.

BROCCOLI & ALMOND MILK SMOOTHIE

155 calories

Ingredients

- 75g/3oz tenderstem broccoli
- 1 nectarine
- 250ml/1 cup unsweetened almond milk
- Ice cubes

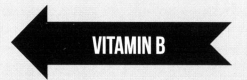

VITAMIN B

Method

1 Rinse the ingredients well.

2 Cut any thick green stalks off the spinach. De-stone the nectarine.

3 Add the fruit & vegetables to the NUTRiBULLET tall cup. Make sure the ingredients do not go past the MAX line on your machine.

4 Add ice, again being careful not to exceed the MAX line.

5 Twist on the NUTRiBULLET blade and blend until smooth.

CHEF'S NOTE

Broccoli contains fibre which help aid digestion.

DOUBLE BERRY SMOOTHIE

195 calories

Ingredients

- 50g/2oz spinach
- 75g/3oz blueberries
- 75g/3oz blackberries
- 3 tbsp low fat vanilla yoghurt
- 1 tsp honey
- Ice Cubes

Method

1 Rinse the ingredients well.

2 Cut any thick green stalks off the spinach.

3 Add the fruit, honey & vegetables to the NUTRiBULLET tall cup. Make sure the ingredients do not go past the MAX line on your machine.

4 Add ice, again being careful not to exceed the MAX line.

5 Twist on the NUTRiBULLET blade and blend until smooth.

CHEF'S NOTE
Any mix of soft berries will work for this simple smoothie

APRICOT & BANANA BLAST

198 calories

Ingredients

- 50g/3oz spinach
- 2 fresh apricots
- 1 banana
- Water

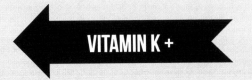

VITAMIN K +

Method

1 Rinse the ingredients well.

2 Cut any thick green stalks off the spinach.

3 Halve and stone the apricots. Peel the banana.

4 Add the fruit & vegetables to the NUTRiBULLET tall cup. Make sure the ingredients do not go past the MAX line on your machine.

5 Add water, again being careful not to exceed the MAX line.

6 Twist on the NUTRiBULLET blade and blend until smooth.

CHEF'S NOTE
Try replacing kale for the spinach.

BLUEBERRY SOYA SMOOTHIE

139 calories

Ingredients

- 75g/3oz fresh blackberry
- 250ml/1 cup soya milk
- A pinch of ground cinnamon
- 1 tsp honey
- Water

Method

1 Rinse the blueberries and place them in the NUTRiBULLET tall cup.

2 Add the cinnamon, honey and soya milk. Make sure the ingredients do not go past the MAX line on your machine.

3 Add a little water if needed to take it up to the MAX line.

4 Twist on the NUTRiBULLET blade and blend until smooth.

CHEF'S NOTE

Blackberries are rich in antioxidants and have anti-bacterial properties which help in cleansing the blood.

BRIGHT CUCUMBER JUICE

155 calories

Ingredients

- 50g/2oz spinach
- ½ cucumber
- 1 tbsp lemon juice
- 1 tbsp flax seed
- Water

Method

1 Rinse the ingredients well.

2 Cut any thick green stalks off the spinach.

3 Nip the end of the cucumber but don't bother peeling it.

4 Add the spinach, cucumber, lemon juice & flax seed to the NUTRiBULLET tall cup. Make sure the ingredients do not go past the MAX line on your machine.

5 Add water, again being careful not to exceed the MAX line.

6 Twist on the NUTRiBULLET blade and blend until smooth.

CHEF'S NOTE
Cucumbers contain vitamin K, B vitamins, copper, potassium, vitamin C, and manganese.

FLAX SEED & CARROT SMOOTHIE

188 calories

Ingredients

- 50g/2oz spinach
- 150g/5oz carrots
- 1 apple

- 2 tsp flax seed
- Water

Method

1 Rinse the ingredients well.

2 Cut any thick green stalks off the spinach.

3 Top & tail the carrots, no need to peel. Core the apple.

4 Add the spinach, apple, carrot & flax seed to the NUTRiBULLET tall cup. Make sure the ingredients do not go past the MAX line on your machine.

5 Add water, again being careful not to exceed the MAX line.

6 Twist on the NUTRiBULLET blade and blend until smooth.

CHEF'S NOTE

Flax seeds are rich in omega 3's.

PEACH PROTEIN PLUS

189 calories

Ingredients

- 1 scoop protein powder, vanilla flavour
- 250ml/1 cup unsweetened almond milk
- 1 peach
- Ice cubes

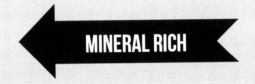

MINERAL RICH

Method

1 Wash, halve and de-stone the peach.

2 Add everything to the NUTRiBULLET tall cup.

3 Make sure the ingredients do not go past the MAX line on your machine.

4 Twist on the NUTRiBULLET blade and blend until smooth.

CHEF'S NOTE
Use whichever flavour of protein powder you prefer.

GOJI BERRY SUPERFOOD SMOOTHIE

196 calories

Ingredients

- 1 tbsp dried goji berries
- 50g/2oz strawberries
- 1 tsp honey
- 250ml/1 cup unsweetened almond milk
- Water
- Ice

Method

1 Soak the goji berries in a little water for around 15 minutes.

2 Rinse the strawberries well and remove the green tops.

3 Place all the berries in the NUTRiBULLET tall cup. Add the honey, almond milk and ice to taste, making sure the ingredients do not go past the MAX line on your machine.

4 Top up with a little water if needed.

5 Twist on the NUTRiBULLET blade and blend until smooth.

CHEF'S NOTE
Goji berries are a wonderful superfood - they're packed with antioxidants, vitamins, minerals and fibre.

COCONUT WATER SPINACH JUICE

156 calories

Ingredients

- 50g/2oz spinach
- 200g/7oz carrots
- 250ml/1 cup coconut water
- 1 tsp honey
- Water

Method

1 Rinse the ingredients well.

2 Cut any thick green stalks off the spinach

3 Top & tail the carrots, no need to peel.

4 Add the vegetables, honey & coconut water to the NUTRiBULLET tall cup. Make sure the ingredients do not go past the MAX line on your machine.

5 Add a little water if needed to take it up to the MAX line.

6 Twist on the NUTRiBULLET blade and blend until smooth.

CHEF'S NOTE
Coconut water contains essential amino acids.

SOYA SPINACH SMOOTHIE

197 calories

Ingredients

LOW FAT

- 50g/2oz spinach
- 1 peach
- 250ml/1 cup unsweetened almond milk
- Water

Method

1 Rinse the ingredients well.

2 Cut any thick green stalks off the spinach.

3 Peel and stone the peach.

4 Add the spinach, peach & almond milk to the NUTRiBULLET tall cup. Make sure the ingredients do not go past the MAX line on your machine.

5 Add a little water if needed to take it up to the MAX line.

6 Twist on the NUTRiBULLET blade and blend until smooth.

CHEF'S NOTE
This is also good with almond milk in place of soya milk.

CARROT ALMOND MILK

Ingredients

- 25g/1oz spinach
- 125g/4oz carrots
- 250ml/1 cup unsweetened almond milk
- 1 tbsp almonds
- Water

Method

1 Rinse the ingredients well.

2 Cut any thick green stalks off the spinach.

3 Top & tail the carrots, no need to peel.

4 Add the vegetables, almond milk & almonds to the NUTRiBULLET tall cup. Make sure the ingredients do not go past the MAX line on your machine.

5 Add a little water if needed to take it up to the MAX line.

6 Twist on the NUTRiBULLET blade and blend until smooth.

CHEF'S NOTE

Almond milk is naturally low in fat and high in vitamins.

CARROT & APPLE JUICE

195 calories

Ingredients

SKIN CLEANSER ➡

- 50g/2oz spinach
- 1 apple
- 200g/7oz carrots
- Water

Method

1 Rinse the ingredients well.

2 Cut any thick green stalks off the spinach.

3 Peel and core the apple.

4 Top & tail the carrots, no need to peel.

5 Add the fruit and vegetables to the NUTRiBULLET tall cup. Make sure the ingredients do not go past the MAX line on your machine.

6 Add water, again being careful not to exceed the MAX line.

7 Twist on the NUTRiBULLET blade and blend until smooth.

CHEF'S NOTE
The apple and carrot are a naturally sweet base for this juice.

PARSLEY & MANGO SMOOTHIE

195 calories

Ingredients

- 50g/2oz kale
- 125g/4oz mango
- 1 banana
- 1 tbsp chopped flat-leaf parsley
- Water

Method

1 Rinse the kale, remove any thick stems and roughly chop.

2 Peel and de-stone the mango. Peel the banana.

3 Add all the ingredients to the NUTRiBULLET tall cup. Make sure they do not go past the MAX line on your machine.

4 Add a little water if needed to take it up to the MAX line.

5 Twist on the NUTRiBULLET blade and blend until smooth.

CHEF'S NOTE

Parsley is a diuretics that can help flush toxins from your body.

GREEN GRAPE FIG JUICE

180 calories

Ingredients

- 3 figs
- 75g/3oz green, seedless grapes
- 75g/3oz baby spinach
- Pinch of ground cinnamon
- Water
- Ice cubes

Method

1 Rinse the grapes & the spinach and place in the NUTRiBULLET tall cup. Scoop out the pink flesh from the figs, and add.

2 Add the cinnamon and water. Top with ice cubes making sure not to pass the MAX line on your machine.

3 Twist on the NUTRiBULLET blade and blend until smooth.

CHEF'S NOTE
Figs are a good source of fibre.

SWEET GREEN TEA JUICE

175 calories

Ingredients

- 250ml/1 cup chilled green tea
- 1 tbsp lemon juice
- 2 tsp agave nectar
- 1 pear
- Ice cubes

Method

1 Rinse, core and quarter the pear, leaving the skin on.

2 Peel and de-seed the lemon.

3 Add all the ingredients except the ice to the NUTRiBULLET tall cup. Add the ice, only as far as the MAX line on your machine.

4 Twist on the NUTRiBULLET blade and blend until smooth.

CHEF'S NOTE
Green tea is packed full of antioxidants.

GREEN HEMP JUICE

185 calories

Ingredients

- 75g/3oz spinach
- 1 yellow pepper
- 1 apple
- 1 stalk celery

- 1 tbsp hemp seeds
- 2 ice cubes
- Water

Method

1 Rinse the spinach, pepper and celery. De-seed the pepper. Core the apple. Roughly chop the celery.

2 Add the vegetable to the NUTRiBULLET tall cup. Add the hemp seeds and a couple of ice cubes. Make sure the ingredients do not go past the MAX line on your machine.

3 Top up with water if needed, as far as the MAX line.

4 Twist on the NUTRiBULLET blade and blend until smooth.

CHEF'S NOTE
Hemp seeds are rich in essential fatty acids.

POMEGRANATE & BERRY SMOOTHIE

189 calories

Ingredients

- 100g/3½oz blueberries
- ½ banana
- 120ml/½ cup pomegranate juice
- Water

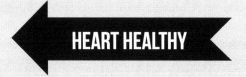

HEART HEALTHY

Method

1 Rinse the blueberries.

2 Peel the banana and break into three pieces. Add them to the NUTRiBULLET tall cup.

3 Add the pomegranate juice, making sure the ingredients do not go past the MAX line on your machine.

4 Add a little water if needed to take it up to the MAX line.

5 Twist on the NUTRiBULLET blade and blend until smooth.

CHEF'S NOTE
Pomegranate is an unexpectedly good source of fibre.

PINEAPPLE SLUSHIE

190 calories

Ingredients

- 1 orange
- ½ kiwi fruit
- 1 banana

- 50g/2oz pineapple
- Water
- Ice cubes

Method

1 Peel the kiwi fruit, banana & pineapple.

2 Peel & de-seed the orange.

3 Add the fruit to the NUTRiBULLET tall cup

4 Add ice and water to taste, making make sure the ingredients do not go past the MAX line on your machine.

5 Twist on the NUTRiBULLET blade and blend until smooth.

CHEF'S NOTE
This is a lovely light and refreshing smoothie.

KIWI JUICE BOOSTER

195 calories

Ingredients

- 1 kiwi
- 1 orange
- 1 apple
- Ice cubes
- Water

Method

1 Rinse the ingredients well.

2 Peel the kiwi. Peel and de-seed the orange.

3 Core the apple.

4 Add the fruit and ice to the NUTRiBULLET tall cup. Make sure the ingredients do not go past the MAX line on your machine.

5 Add water, again being careful not to exceed the MAX line.

6 Twist on the NUTRiBULLET blade and blend until smooth.

CHEF'S NOTE

With its fruit combo, this juice delivers triple Vitamin C goodness.

THE *Skinny*

NUTRiBULLET

LEAN BODY HiiT PLAN

NUTRIBLASTS UNDER 300 CALORIES

GRAPEFRUIT & APPLE JUICE

285 calories

Ingredients

- 50g/2oz spinach
- 1 apple
- 1 grapefruit

- 120ml/½ cup unsweetened almond milk
- Water

Method

1 Rinse and core the apple.

2 Peel and de-seed the grapefruit.

3 Add everything to the NUTRiBULLET tall cup. Top up with ice cubes and water.

4 Make sure the ingredients do not go past the MAX line on your machine.

5 Twist on the NUTRiBULLET blade and blend until smooth.

CHEF'S NOTE

Grapefruit contains natural acids that cleanse the skin as well as vitamin C which acts as an antioxidant.

CHIA CINNAMON SMOOTHIE

210 calories

Ingredients

- 75g/3oz blueberries
- 1 banana
- 2 tsp chia seeds

- ½ tsp ground cinnamon
- 2 tsp honey
- Water

Method

1 Rinse the blueberries well. Peel the banana.

2 Add these to the NUTRiBULLET tall cup, along with the chia seeds, cinnamon and honey. Make sure they don't go past the MAX line on your machine.

3 Top up with water as far as the MAX line.

4 Twist on the NUTRiBULLET blade and blend until smooth.

CHEF'S NOTE
Cinnamon has been used throughout the ages to treat everything from a common cold to muscle spasms.

KALE & AVOCADO SMOOTHIE

296 calories

Ingredients

- 1 banana
- 50g/2oz kale
- ½ ripe avocado
- 1 tsp honey
- Water

Method

1 Peel the banana.

2 Rinse the kale and remove any thick stalks.

3 Peel and stone the avocado.

4 Place all the ingredients in the NUTRiBULLET tall cup, making sure they do not go past the MAX line on your machine.

5 Add a little water if needed to take it up to the MAX line.

6 Twist on the NUTRiBULLET blade and blend until smooth.

CHEF'S NOTE
Avocado and banana create a lovely thick base for this smoothie.

ALMOND PASSION SMOOTHIE

260 calories

Ingredients

- 200g/7oz mango
- 100g/3½oz passion fruit
- 2 tbsp fat-free yoghurt

- 250ml/1 cup unsweetened almond milk
- Water

Method

1 Peel, de-stone and cube the mango. Drop it in the NUTRiBULLET tall cup. Halve the passion fruit and scoop out the flesh, adding it to the cup.

2 Add the other ingredients. Make sure they do not go past the MAX line on your machine.

3 Add a little water if needed to take it up to the MAX line.

4 Twist on the NUTRiBULLET blade and blend until smooth.

CHEF'S NOTE

Try with flavoured yoghurt if you wish.

SWEET KALE JUICE

240 calories

Ingredients

- 2 tsp honey
- 75g/3oz kale
- 200g/7oz pineapple
- 1 apple
- Water

Method

1 Rinse the ingredients well.

2 Cut any thick stalks off the kale.

3 Peel the pineapple. Core the apple.

4 Add the kale, fruit & honey to the NUTRiBULLET tall cup. Make sure the ingredients do not go past the MAX line on your machine.

5 Add water, again being careful not to exceed the MAX line.

6 Twist on the NUTRiBULLET blade and blend until smooth.

CHEF'S NOTE
Low in calories, high in fibre and with zero fat, kale is a mega-smoothie super-food.

TOTALLY TROPICAL

280 calories

Ingredients

- 150g/5oz mango
- 150g/5oz pineapple
- 1 banana
- 1 tbsp Greek yoghurt
- Ice

Method

1 Peel the pineapple and banana.

2 Peel & de-stone the mango.

3 Add the fruit to the NUTRiBULLET tall cup. Make sure the ingredients do not go past the MAX line on your machine.

4 Add ice, again being careful not to exceed the MAX line.

5 Twist on the NUTRiBULLET blade and blend until smooth.

CHEF'S NOTE
You could try making with soya milk too.

NUTTY SWEET POTATO SMOOTHIE

270 calories

Ingredients

- 50g/2oz spinach
- 150g/5oz sweet potato
- 250ml/1 cup unsweetened almond milk
- 1 tbsp almonds
- Water

Method

1 Rinse the ingredients well.

2 Remove any thick stalks from the spinach.

3 Cube the sweet potato, no need to peel.

4 Add the spinach, sweet potato, almond milk & almonds to the NUTRiBULLET tall cup. Make sure the ingredients do not go past the MAX line on your machine.

5 Add a little water if needed to take it up to the MAX line.

6 Twist on the NUTRiBULLET blade and blend until smooth.

CHEF'S NOTE
Sweet potatoes are an exceptionally rich source of vitamin A.

PROTEIN SCOOP SMOOTHIE

290 calories

Ingredients

- 2 tsp flax seeds
- 125g/4oz raspberries
- 1 scoop vanilla protein powder
- 250ml/1 cup semi skimmed milk
- Ice cubes

Method

1 Rinse the raspberries and add everything to the NUTRiBULLET tall cup, finishing with ice. Make sure the ice does not go past the MAX line on your machine.

2 Twist on the NUTRiBULLET blade and blend until smooth.

CHEF'S NOTE

Flax seeds can help eliminate toxins from the body, regulate the metabolism and reduce blood sugar levels.

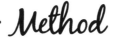

SALAD SPICE JUICE

255 calories

Ingredients

- 1 tomato
- ½ cucumber
- ½ clove garlic
- 1 stalk celery
- 1 small romaine lettuce
- ½ avocado

- ¼ tsp turmeric
- 1 tbsp lemon juice
- 1 tbsp chopped fresh mint leaves
- 1 tsp ground ginger
- 1 pinch cayenne pepper
- Ice

Method

1 Rinse the ingredients well. Roughly chop the cucumber, celery and lettuce.

2 Peel the garlic and avocado. De-stone the avocado.

3 Add everything to the NUTRiBULLET tall cup, finishing with ice. Make sure the ingredients do not go past the MAX line on your machine.

4 Twist on the NUTRiBULLET blade and blend until smooth.

CHEF'S NOTE
Ginger has a long history of use for treating nausea, motion sickness and pain.

PEAR & SOYA SMOOTHIE

288 calories

Ingredients

- 1 pear
- 1 banana
- 120ml/½ cup soya milk

- 2 tbsp natural low-fat yoghurt
- 2 tsp flax seeds

Method

1 Rinse and core the pear.

2 Peel the banana and break into three.

3 Place them in the NUTRiBULLET tall cup. Add the milk, yoghurt and flax seeds. Make sure the ingredients do not go past the MAX line on your machine.

4 Twist on the NUTRiBULLET blade and blend until smooth.

CHEF'S NOTE
Pears contain pectin that has a positive mild laxative effect on the body.

GINGER SPICED ORANGE JUICE

255 calories

Ingredients

- 250ml/1 cup freshly squeezed orange juice
- 1 apple
- 2 tsp grated fresh ginger
- 50g/2oz spinach
- Ice cubes

Method

1 Rinse the apple and the spinach. Core and chop the apple.

2 Add all the ingredients to the NUTRiBULLET tall cup, finishing with ice cubes to taste. Make sure the ingredients do not go past the MAX line on your machine.

3 Twist on the NUTRiBULLET blade and blend until smooth.

CHEF'S NOTE
High in antioxidants, nutrients and vitamin C, fresh orange juice is a great detox ingredient.

RASPBERRY FLAX SMOOTHIE

220 calories

Ingredients

- 125g/4oz raspberries
- 1 tbsp flax seeds
- 50g/2oz spinach

- 2 tbsp low fat Greek yogurt
- 250ml/1 cup coconut water
- Water

Method

1 Wash the spinach and raspberries well and place them in the NUTRiBULLET tall cup.

2 Add the flax seeds, yoghurt and coconut water. Make sure they don't go past the MAX line on your machine.

3 Top up with water as far as the MAX line.

4 Twist on the NUTRiBULLET blade and blend until smooth.

CHEF'S NOTE
Flax seeds are rich in protein and fibre.

VIT C + SMOOTHIE MILK

230 calories

Ingredients

- 125g/4oz mango
- ½ banana
- 120ml/½ cup soya milk

- 50g/2oz pineapple
- 120ml/½ cup orange juice
- Water

Method

1 Peel and de-stone the mango.

2 Peel the banana and the pineapple.

3 Add everything to the NUTRiBULLET tall cup, making sure the ingredients do not go past the MAX line on your machine.

4 Add a little water if needed to take it up to the MAX line.

5 Twist on the NUTRiBULLET blade and blend until smooth.

CHEF'S NOTE
For extra creaminess, use a whole banana. Your smoothie will still be less than 300 calories.

WATERMELON & CHIA SEED SMOOTHIE

280 calories

Ingredients

- 250g/9oz watermelon
- 1 tbsp chia seeds
- 1 apple
- 250ml/1 cup unsweetened almond milk
- 1 tsp honey
- Water
- Ice

Method

1 Scoop out the watermelon flesh, de-seed and place in the NUTRiBULLET tall cup.

2 Core the apple.

3 Add all the other ingredients, finishing with ice as far as the MAX line on your machine.

4 Twist on the NUTRiBULLET blade and blend until smooth.

CHEF'S NOTE

Watermelon is believed to have the most potent cancer-fighting properties of any fruit.

COCONUT & PINEAPPLE GREEN SMOOTHIE

240 calories

Ingredients

- 50g/2oz kale
- 250ml/1 cup coconut water
- 1 banana
- 2 tbsp low fat natural yogurt
- 75g/3oz fresh pineapple
- Water

Method

1 Rinse the kale well and remove any thick stalks.

2 Peel the banana and break into three pieces. Peel the pineapple.

3 Add all the ingredients the to the NUTRiBULLET tall cup. Make sure they do not go past the MAX line on your machine.

4 Add a little water if needed to take it up to the MAX line.

5 Twist on the NUTRiBULLET blade and blend until smooth.

CHEF'S NOTE
Use tinned pineapple if you don't have fresh pineapple to hand.

SMOOTH SUPER GREEN SMOOTHIE

285 calories

Ingredients

- 50g/2oz kale
- 50g/1oz spinach
- ½ avocado
- 1 tsp honey

- 1 apple
- Water
- Ice cubes

Method

1 Wash the kale & spinach. Cut any thick stems off the kale.

2 Peel and de-stone the avocado. Core the apple.

3 Place everything in the NUTRiBULLET tall cup and add some ice cubes . Make sure the ingredients do not go past the MAX line on your machine.

4 Add a little water if needed.

5 Twist on the NUTRiBULLET blade and blend until smooth.

CHEF'S NOTE
Kale is nutrient-rich and contains zero fat.

MANGO YOGHURT SMOOTHIE

Ingredients

- 125g/4oz mango
- 4 tbsp natural low-fat Greek yogurt
- 250ml/1 cup unsweetened almond milk
- 1 tsp honey
- Water

Method

1 Peel and de-stone the mango.

2 Add to the NUTRiBULLET tall cup, along with the other ingredients.

3 Make sure the ingredients do not go past the MAX line on your machine.

4 Add a little water if needed to take it up to the MAX line.

5 Twist on the NUTRiBULLET blade and blend until smooth.

CHEF'S NOTE
Make sure your mango is ripe for maximum sweetness!

APRICOT ALMOND MILK

245 calories

Ingredients

 VITAMIN A

- 2 apricots
- 1 banana
- 250ml/1 cup unsweetened almond milk
- Ice

Method

1 Rinse, halve and de-stone the apricot.

2 Peel the banana.

3 Add fruit to the NUTRiBULLET tall cup. Pour in the milk and add ice to taste. Make sure the ingredients do not go past the MAX line on your machine.

4 Twist on the NUTRiBULLET blade and blend until smooth.

CHEF'S NOTE
For a creamier finish add some Greek yoghurt.

PEAR & BANANA CINNAMON SMOOTHIE

275 calories

Ingredients

- 1 pear
- 1 banana
- 120ml/½ cup semi-skimmed milk
- 2 tbsp low fat yoghurt
- 1 large pinch ground cinnamon

Method

1 Rinse, core and quarter the pear, leaving the skin on.

2 Peel the banana.

3 Add the fruit to the NUTRiBULLET tall cup followed by the other ingredients, making sure not to go past the MAX line on your machine.

4 Add a little water if needed to take it up to the MAX line.

5 Twist on the NUTRiBULLET blade and blend until smooth.

CHEF'S NOTE
As an alternative, try using light coconut milk instead of semi-skimmed milk.

THE *Skinny*
NUTRiBULLET
LEAN BODY HiiT PLAN
NUTRIBLASTS UNDER 400 CALORIES

COCONUT MILK MINT SMOOTHIE

365 calories

Ingredients

- 1 shredded romaine lettuce
- 1 apple
- 1 tbsp lemon juice
- ¼ cucumber
- 1 tbsp chopped fresh mint
- 250ml/1 cup low fat coconut milk

Method

1 Rinse the ingredients well.

2 Core the apple, leaving the skin on. Peel the lemon; don't worry about removing the pips.

3 Dice the cucumber, leaving the skin on.

4 Add all the ingredients to the NUTRiBULLET tall cup. Making sure they do not go past the MAX line on your machine.

5 Twist on the NUTRiBULLET blade and blend until smooth.

CHEF'S NOTE
Add some water if you want to fill up to the max line.

MORNING GLORY AVOCADO SMOOTHIE

389 calories

Ingredients

- 50g/2oz spinach
- ½ ripe avocado
- 1 apple

- 1 banana
- 2 tsp pumpkin seeds
- Water

Method

1 Rinse the ingredients well.

2 Scoop out the avocado flesh discarding the rind & stone.

3 Core the apple, leaving the skin on. Peel the banana and break into three pieces.

4 Add the fruit, vegetables & flax seeds to the NUTRiBULLET tall cup. Make sure the ingredients do not go past the MAX line on your machine.

5 Add water, again being careful not to exceed the MAX line.

6 Twist on the NUTRiBULLET blade and blend until smooth.

CHEF'S NOTE
Try flax seeds as an alternative to pumpkin seeds.

MELON & CASHEW GREEN SMOOTHIE

360 calories

Ingredients

- 50g/2oz spinach
- 1 apple
- 200g/7oz cantaloupe melon
- 250ml/1 cup semi skimmed milk
- 1 tbsp cashew nuts
- Water

Method

1 Rinse the ingredients well.

2 Core the apple, leaving the skin on.

3 Scoop out the melon flesh, discarding the seeds & rind.

4 Add the fruit, vegetables & nuts to the NUTRiBULLET tall cup. Make sure the ingredients do not go past the MAX line on your machine.

5 Add water, again being careful not to exceed the MAX line.

6 Twist on the NUTRiBULLET blade and blend until smooth.

CHEF'S NOTE
Try almonds or walnuts in place of the cashew nuts.

HONEY WALNUT SMOOTHIE

375 calories

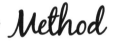
Ingredients

- 1 orange
- 200g/7oz mixed berries
- 250ml/1 cup unsweetened almond milk
- 1 tsp honey
- 8 walnuts halves
- Water

Method

1 Rinse the ingredients well.

2 Peel the orange and separate into segments.

3 Add the fruit, milk, honey & walnuts to the NUTRiBULLET tall cup. Make sure the ingredients do not go past the MAX line on your machine.

4 Add water, again being careful not to exceed the MAX line.

5 Twist on the NUTRiBULLET blade and blend until smooth.

CHEF'S NOTE
The fresh walnuts should be shelled before adding to the cup.

GINGER BEETROOT FRUIT JUICE

305 calories

Ingredients

- 50g/2oz spinach
- 1 fresh medium beetroot
- 1 pear
- 1 apple
- 125g/4oz strawberries
- 2cm/1 inch fresh ginger root
- Water

Method

1 Rinse the ingredients well.

2 Remove any thick stalks from the spinach.

3 Cut the green stalks off the beetroot and dice.

4 Core the apple & pear, leave the skin on.

5 Add all the fruit & vegetables to the NUTRiBULLET tall cup. Make sure the ingredients do not go past the MAX line on your machine.

6 Add water, again being careful not to exceed the MAX line.

7 Twist on the NUTRiBULLET blade and blend until smooth.

CHEF'S NOTE
Optional Nutriboost: Add 1 teaspoon flax seeds.

FRUITY OAT SMOOTHIE

320 calories

Ingredients

- 125g/4oz strawberries
- 1 banana
- 250ml/1 cup unsweetened almond milk
- 2 tbsp rolled oats
- Water

Method

1 Rinse the strawberries well and nip off the green tops.

2 Peel the banana.

3 Add all the ingredients to the NUTRiBULLET tall cup. Make sure the ingredients do not go past the MAX line on your machine.

4 Add a little more water if needed to take it up to the MAX line.

5 Twist on the NUTRiBULLET blade and blend until smooth.

CHEF'S NOTE
Strawberries are great for cleansing due to the antioxidants and fibre.

CHOCOLATE RASPBERRY SOYA MILK

325 calories

Ingredients

- 1 banana
- 1 tbsp dark cocoa powder
- 250ml/1 cup soya milk
- 125g/4oz raspberries
- Ice

Method

1 Peel the banana.

2 Rinse the strawberries and remove the green tops.

3 Place them in the NUTRiBULLET tall cup, together with the coconut milk and cocoa powder. Add ice, but make sure it doesn't go past the MAX line on your machine.

4 Twist on the NUTRiBULLET blade and blend until smooth.

CHEF'S NOTE
Dark cocoa contains antioxidants that regular cocoa doesn't have.

ALMOND & MANGO SMOOTHIE

355 calories

Ingredients

- 200g/7oz mango
- 1 banana
- 250ml/1 cup unsweetened almond milk
- 1 tbsp almonds
- Water

Method

1 Peel, stone and cube the mango.

2 Peel the banana.

3 Add everything to the NUTRiBULLET tall cup. Make sure the ingredients do not go past the MAX line on your machine.

4 Twist on the NUTRiBULLET blade and blend until smooth.

CHEF'S NOTE

Bananas are rich in fibre, vitamins B6, and minerals like potassium and manganese, which make them very nutritious and great for detox.

CREAMY PARSLEY & AVOCADO BLEND

330 calories

Ingredients

- ¼ cucumber
- 1 tbsp fresh flat leaf parsley
- 50g/2oz spinach

- ½ ripe avocado,
- 180ml/¾ cup light coconut milk
- Ice cubes

Method

1 Rinse the cucumber, parsley and spinach. Roughly chop the cucumber. Peel and de-stone the avocado.

2 Add all the ingredients to the NUTRiBULLET tall cup, finishing with ice to taste, but make sure you do not go past the MAX line on your machine.

3 Twist on the NUTRiBULLET blade and blend until smooth.

CHEF'S NOTE
Parsley is rich in many vital vitamins, including Vitamin C, B 12, K and A.

TOMATO KALE SMOOTHIE

305 calories

Ingredients

- 1 apple
- ¼ cucumber
- 1 tbsp flax seeds
- 2 tomatoes

- 50g/2oz kale
- 250ml/1 cup unsweetened almond milk
- Water

Method

1 Rinse the kale, cucumber & apple.

2 Core the apple. Roughly chop the cucumber and remove the thick stalks from the kale

3 Put all the ingredients except water into the NUTRiBULLET tall cup. Make sure they do not go past the MAX line on your machine.

4 Add a little water if needed to take it up to the MAX line.

5 Twist on the NUTRiBULLET blade and blend until smooth.

CHEF'S NOTE
Flaxseeds are a rich source of micro-nutrients, dietary fibre, manganese, vitamin B1, and the essential fatty acid omega-3.

DOUBLE BERRY JUICE

305 calories

Ingredients

- 50g/2oz spinach
- 1 banana
- 125g/4oz mixed berries
- 125g/4oz fresh peeled pineapple
- Small pinch ground cinnamon
- Water

Method

1 Rinse the ingredients well.

2 Remove any thick stalks from the spinach.

3 Peel the banana and break into three pieces.

4 Add the fruit, vegetables & ground cinnamon to the NUTRiBULLET tall cup. Make sure the ingredients do not go past the MAX line on your machine.

5 Add water, again being careful not to exceed the MAX line.

6 Twist on the NUTRiBULLET blade and blend until smooth.

CHEF'S NOTE
Feel free to experiment with the cinnamon quantity in this recipe - you may prefer a little more.

NUTMEG PINEAPPLE CLEANSE

320 calories

Ingredients

- 1 banana
- 125g/4oz carrots
- 120ml/½ cup light coconut milk
- 100g/3½oz pineapple
- ¼ tsp ground nutmeg

Method

1 Peel the banana and pineapple.

2 Top and tail and peel the carrots.

3 Add everything to the NUTRiBULLET tall cup. Make sure the ingredients do not go past the MAX line on your machine.

4 Add a little water if needed to take it up to the MAX line.

5 Twist on the NUTRiBULLET blade and blend until smooth.

CHEF'S NOTE

Nutmeg increases immune system function.

ORANGE GINGER JUICE

325 calories

Ingredients

- 1 orange
- 1 apple
- 2cm/1 inch fresh peeled ginger
- 1 tbsp honey
- 2 tbsp low fat yoghurt
- 1 banana
- 1 tbsp lemon juice
- Water

Method

1 Peel and de-seed the orange.

2 Finely grate the ginger.

3 Peel the banana and break into three pieces.

4 Add everything to the tall cup. Make sure the ingredients do not go past the MAX line on your machine.

5 Add a little water if needed to take it up to the MAX line.

6 Twist on the NUTRiBULLET blade and blend until smooth.

CHEF'S NOTE
Ginger is prized for it's healing and detoxifying properties.

GREEN SOYA PUMPKIN MILK

330 calories

Ingredients

- 1 pear
- 1 apple
- 50g/2oz spinach
- 250ml/1 cup soya milk
- 1 tbsp pumpkin seeds
- Water

Method

1 Wash the spinach and the pear. Core the pear and apple but don't peel them.

2 Add all the ingredients except water to the NUTRiBULLET tall cup. Make sure they do not go past the MAX line on your machine.

3 Add a little water if needed to take it up to the MAX line.

4 Twist on the NUTRiBULLET blade and blend until smooth.

CHEF'S NOTE
Pumpkin seeds provide heart-healthy magnesium.

GOJI BERRY COCONUT BLASTER

380 calories

Ingredients

- 250ml/1 cup coconut water
- 1 tbsp coconut cream
- ½ ripe avocado
- 3 tbsp low fat natural yogurt
- 100g/3½oz strawberries
- 1 tbsp goji berries
- Water

Method

1 Rinse the strawberries and remove the green tops.

2 Peel & de-stone the avocado.

3 Add all the ingredients to the NUTRiBULLET tall cup. Make sure they don't go past the MAX line on your machine.

4 Twist on the NUTRiBULLET blade and blend until smooth.

CHEF'S NOTE
Soak goji berries in warm water for a few minutes before using.

CASHEW & COCONUT MILK SMOOTHIE

340 calories

Ingredients

GOOD FATS →

- 10 cashew nuts
- 75g/3oz spinach
- 250ml/1 cup light coconut milk
- Ice cubes

Method

1 Rinse the spinach well.

2 Add all the ingredients to the NUTRiBULLET tall cup, finishing with ice. Make sure they do not go past the MAX line on your machine.

3 Twist on the NUTRiBULLET blade and blend until smooth.

CHEF'S NOTE
Vary the quantity of nuts to suit your own taste but be aware of the calorie count if you do this.

MINT & CHIA GREEN SMOOTHIE

310 calories

Ingredients

- 75g/3oz spinach
- 1 banana
- ¼ ripe avocado
- 1 tbsp chopped fresh mint

- 2 tsp chia seeds
- 250ml/1 cup unsweetened almond milk
- Water

Method

1 Rinse the spinach. Peel the banana. Peel and de-stone the avocado.

2 Add everything to the NUTRiBULLET tall cup. Make sure the ingredients do not go past the MAX line on your machine.

3 Add a little water if needed to take it up to the MAX line.

4 Twist on the NUTRiBULLET blade and blend until smooth.

CHEF'S NOTE
Chia seeds can help raise HDL cholesterol – which is the good cholesterol that helps protect against heart attack and stroke.

DATE & BANANA SMOOTHIE

320 calories

Ingredients

- 1 banana
- 4 pitted dates
- ¼ ripe avocado
- 250ml/1 cup unsweetened almond milk
- Large pinch ground cinnamon

Method

1 Peel the banana. Halve the dates.

2 Peel and stone the avocado.

3 Add everything to the NUTRiBULLET tall cup. Make sure the ingredients do not go past the MAX line on your machine.

4 Twist on the NUTRiBULLET blade and blend until smooth.

CHEF'S NOTE

Feel free to add more almond milk as far as the MAX line if you wish, but remember it will increase your calorie intake.

APPLE GREEN SMOOTHIE

330 calories

Ingredients

- 1 banana
- 1 apple
- 150g/5oz seedless green grapes
- 4 tbsp low fat vanilla yoghurt
- 50g/2oz fresh spinach
- Water

Method

1 Rinse the spinach, grapes and apple.

2 Core the apple and peel the banana.

3 Add all the ingredients to the NUTRiBULLET tall cup. Make sure they do not go past the MAX line on your machine.

4 Add a little water if needed to take it up to the MAX line.

5 Twist on the NUTRiBULLET blade and blend until smooth.

CHEF'S NOTE
Natural yoghurt instead of vanilla also works well.

HiiT Plan WORKOUTS

High Intensity Interval Training is a super fast and really effective way to workout. The short but intense bursts of exercise with rest in between makes your heart work harder and so increases cardio strength, improves metabolism and as a result helps your body burn more calories both during and after your workout. HiiT can also help control blood sugar levels.

It's a very efficient way to train to build a leaner, fitter body and because no equipment is required you can workout at home or just about anywhere.

We have compiled **4** core workouts to perform throughout each week. Choose one workout to perform per day and use the remaining 3 days to rest. Try to alternate between training and rest days. Each workout lasts for approximately 15 mins and a simple explanation of how to correctly perform each exercise in the set is explained in the following pages.

It's very important to warm up your muscles and joints before beginning any exercise to prevent injury and to make sure you perform each repetition to the best of your ability. Stretch for at least 2 minutes before your workout (see page 94 for stretches), then warm up by jogging on the spot for two minutes.

Always cool down and stretch again at the end of your workout.

Tips

- Warm up and cool down before and after each workout
- Have a bottle of water to drink from between sets
- Remember to breathe through each exercise
- Keep your core tight & give maximum effort
- Focus on maintaining correct posture & form for each exercise

HiiT WORKOUT ONE

- Exercise 1: **HIGH KNEES** 20 secs | 10 secs rest
- Exercise 2: **BODYWEIGHT SQUATS** 20 secs | 10 secs rest
- Exercise 3: **JUMPING JACKS** 20 secs | 10 secs rest
- Exercise 4: **SIDE LUNGE** 20 secs | 10 secs rest
- Exercise 5: **TRICEP DIPS** 20 secs | 10 secs rest
- Exercise 6: **MOUNTAIN CLIMBERS** 20 secs | 10 sec rest
- Exercise 7: **BUTT KICKS** 20 secs | 2 minute rest

Repeat for 2 more sets

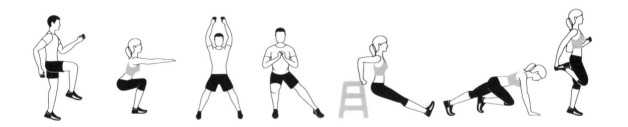

Perform each exercise as many times as possible within 20 seconds. Rest for 10 seconds then perform the next exercise again for 20 secs with a 10 sec rest in between exercises. Repeat until all 7 exercises have been completed.

Rest for 2 minutes then repeat the whole set two more times with a 2 minute rest in between.

Remember that these are high intensity workouts so try to push yourself to get as many repetitions of each exercise with the correct form within the 20 second period.

High KNEES

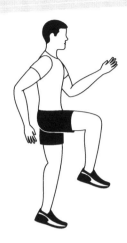 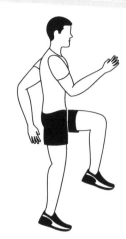

Stand straight with the feet hip width apart, looking straight ahead and arms hanging down by your side. Jump from one foot to the other at the same time lifting your knees as high as possible, hip height is advisable. The arms should be following the motion. Try holding your hands just above the hips so that your knees touch the palms of your hands as you lift your knees.

Bodyweight SQUATS

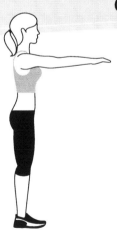 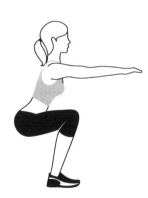

Stand with your feet shoulder width apart with your arms extended in front of you. Begin the movement by flexing your knees and hips, sitting back with your hips until your thighs are parallel with the floor in the full squat position. Quickly reverse the motion until you return to the starting position. As you keep your head and chest up.

Jumping JACKS

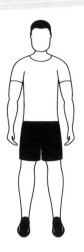 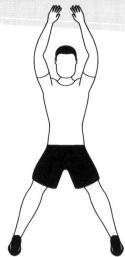

Stand with your feet together and your hands down by your side. In one motion jump your feet out to the side and raise your arms above your head. Immediately reverse by jumping back to the starting position.

Side LUNGE

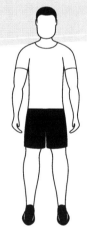 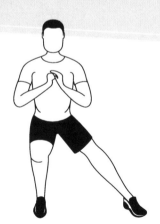

Stand with your knees and hips slightly bent, feet shoulder-width apart and the head and chest up. Keeping your left leg straight, step out to the side with your right leg and bend at your right knee transferring weight to your right side. Extend through the right leg to return to the starting position. Repeat on the left leg.

Tricep DIPS

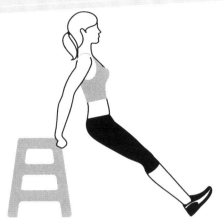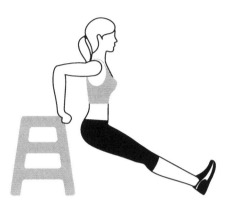

Position your hands shoulder-width apart on a secure bench or stable chair. Slide off the front of the bench with your legs extended out in front of you. Straighten your arms, keeping a slight bend in your elbows. Slowly bend your elbows to lower your body toward the floor until your elbows are at about a 90-degree angle. At this point press down into the bench or chair to straighten your elbows, returning to the starting position.

Mountain CLIMBER

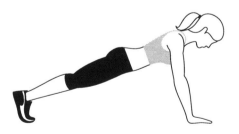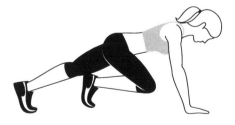

Begin in a pushup position, with your weight supported by your hands and toes. Flexing the knee and hip, bring one leg towards the corresponding arm. Explosively reverse the positions of your legs, extending the bent leg until the leg is straight and supported by the toe, and bringing the other foot up with the hip and knee flexed. Repeat in an alternating fashion.

Butt KICKS

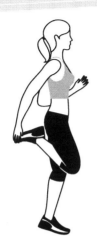 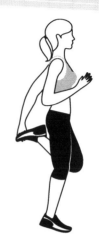

Stand with your legs shoulder-width apart and your arms bent. Flex the right knee and kick your right heel up toward your glutes. Bring the right foot back down while flexing your left knee and kicking your left foot up toward your glutes. Repeat in a continuous movement.

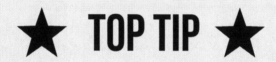

Warm up properly. By warming up your muscles you will reduce the chances of injury or strain. Warm up with jogging on the spot, gentle jumping jacks and stretches (see page 94) for at least 2 minutes.

HiiT WORKOUT TWO

- Exercise 1: **BURPEES** 20 secs | 10 secs rest
- Exercise 2: **JAB SQUATS** 20 secs | 10 secs rest
- Exercise 3: **MUMMY KICKS** 20 secs | 10 secs rest
- Exercise 4: **SIDE SKATER** 20 secs | 10 secs rest
- Exercise 5: **TUCK JUMP** 20 secs | 10 secs rest
- Exercise 6: **SPRINTS** 20 secs | 10 sec rest
- Exercise 7: **HEISMAN** 20 secs | 2 minute rest

Repeat for 2 more sets

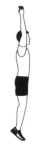 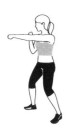 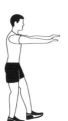 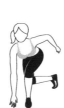 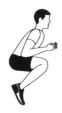 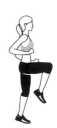 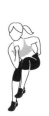

Perform each exercise as many times as possible within 20 seconds. Rest for 10 seconds then perform the next exercise again for 20 secs with a 10 sec rest in between exercises. Repeat until all 7 exercises have been completed.

Rest for 2 minutes then repeat the whole set two more times with a 2 minute rest in between.

Remember that these are high intensity workouts so try to push yourself to get as many repetitions of each exercise with the correct form within the 20 second period.

Burpees

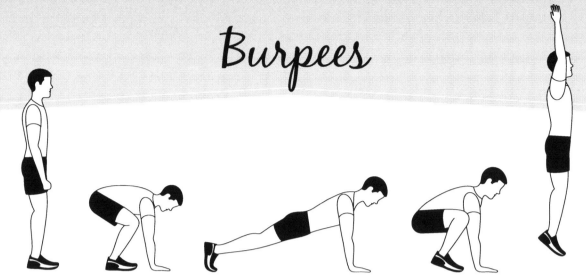

Stand with your feet shoulder-width apart, with your arms at your sides. Push your hips back, bend your knees, and lower your body into a squat before placing your hands on the floor directly in front of, and just inside, your feet. Jump your feet back to land in a plank position forming a straight line from head to toe with a straight back. Jump your feet back again so that they land just outside of your hands. Reach your arms over head and explosively jump up into the air. Land and immediately lower back into a squat for your next repetition.

Jab SQUATS

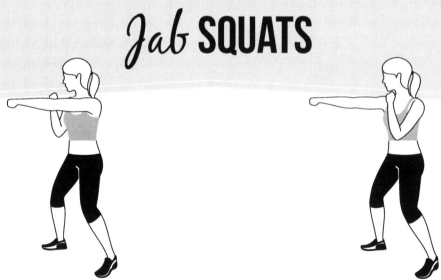

Start in a half squat position with your feet shoulder-width apart and knees slightly bent. Bring your arms up so the palms are facing the sides of your face. Clench your fists. Use sharp movements to lengthen your right arm in front in a punching motion then return to the starting position immediately punching out your left arm. Keep switching sides in a quick powerful motion.

Mummy KICKS

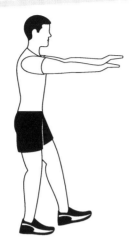 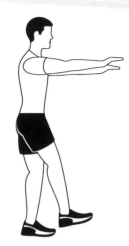

Begin by standing with your arms extended straight out in front. Perform light hop kicks with your feet while simultaneously criss-crossing your hands. Alternate the motion of your arms and hands as you swap between legs. Keep your core tight.

Side SKATER

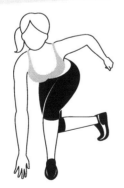 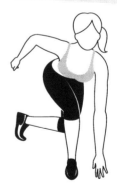

Start in a squat position with your left leg bent at the knee and your right arm parallel for balance. Your right leg is extended but still bent at the knee behind you. Jump sideways to the right, landing on your right leg. Bring your left leg behind you with your left arm extended and fingers touching the floor. Keep your back straight and your core engaged. Reverse direction by jumping to the left.

Tuck JUMP

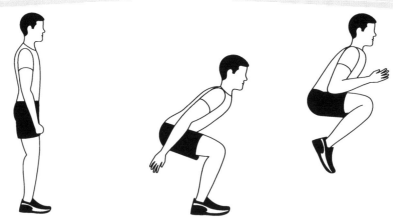

Begin in a standing position with knees slightly bent and arms at your sides. Bend your knees and lower your body quickly into a squat position, then explosively jump upwards bringing your knees up towards your chest.

Sprints

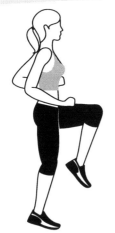 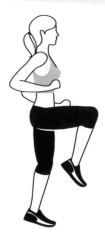

Standing with your feet shoulder-width apart, move your arms and torso as though you are running as fast as you can on the spot. Move feet and legs as little as possible avoiding twisting from side to side.

Heisman

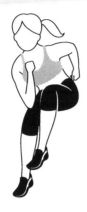 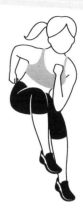

Begin by standing with feet shoulder-width apart and knees slightly bent. Jump onto your right foot while pulling your left knee up and towards the left shoulder. Next jump onto your left foot while pulling your right knee towards the right shoulder. Continue the movement in a quick motion, switching between legs.

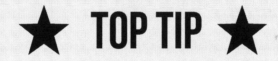

Use a timer or stopwatch to precisely time each exercise and your rest time. There are many free apps available online. Try searching for 'tabata timer app'.

HiiT WORKOUT THREE

- Exercise 1: **SIT UPS** 20 secs | 10 secs rest
- Exercise 2: **BICYCLE CRUNCH** 20 secs | 10 secs rest
- Exercise 3: **MUMMY KICKS** 20 secs | 10 secs rest
- Exercise 4: **JAB SQUATS** 20 secs | 10 secs rest
- Exercise 5: **LATERALS** 20 secs | 10 secs rest
- Exercise 6: **MOUNTAIN CLIMBER** 20 secs | 10 sec rest
- Exercise 7: **TAP UP** 20 secs | 2 minute rest

Repeat for 2 more sets

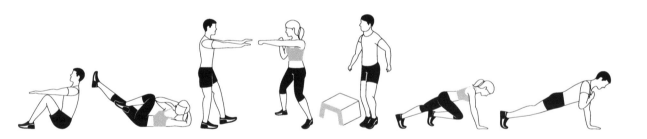

Perform each exercise as many times as possible within 20 seconds. Rest for 10 seconds then perform the next exercise again for 20 secs with a 10 sec rest in between exercises. Repeat until all 7 exercises have been completed.

Rest for 2 minutes then repeat the whole set two more times with a 2 minute rest in between.

Remember that these are high intensity workouts so try to push yourself to get as many repetitions of each exercise with the correct form within the 20 second period.

Sit UPS

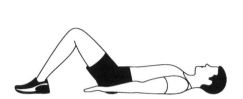 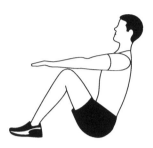

Lie on your back with your knees bent and your arms extended at your sides. and your feet flat on the floor. Engage your core and slowly curl your upper back off the floor towards your knees with your arms extended out. Roll back down to the starting position.

Bicycle CRUNCH

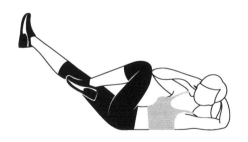 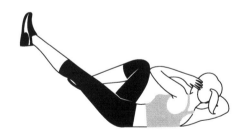

Lie face up and place your hands at the side of your head (do not pull on the back of your head). Make sure your core is tight and the small of your back is pushed hard against the floor. Lift your knees in toward your chest while lifting your shoulder blades off the floor. Rotate to the right, bringing the left elbow towards the right knee as you extend the other leg into the air. Switch sides, bringing the right elbow towards the left knee. Alternate each side in a pedaling motion..

Mummy KICKS

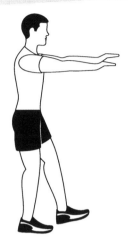 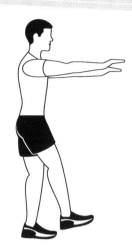

Begin by standing with your arms extended straight out in front. Perform light hop kicks with your feet while simultaneously criss-crossing your hands. Alternate the motion of your arms and hands as you swap between legs. Keep your core tight.

Jab SQUATS

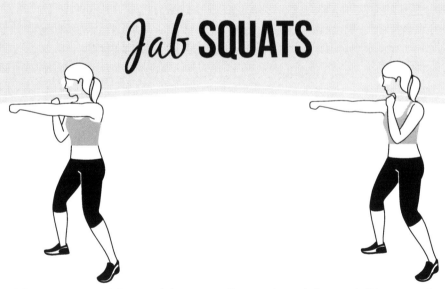

Start in a half squat position with your feet shoulder-width apart and knees slightly bent. Bring your arms up so the palms are facing the sides of your face. Clench your fists. Use sharp movements to lengthen your right arm in front in a punching motion then return to the starting position immediately punching out your left arm. Keep switching sides in a quick powerful motion.

Laterals

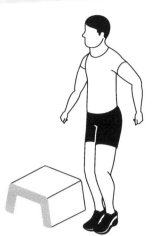 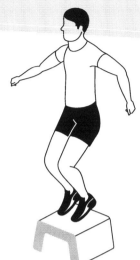

Stand beside a step or box. Position into a quarter squat then jump up and over to the right landing on the box with both feet landing together. Bring your knees high enough to ensure your feet clear the box. Jump over to the other side and repeat, this time jumping to the left.

Mountain CLIMBER

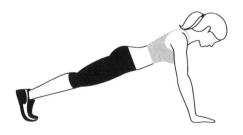 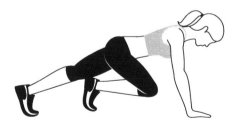

Begin in a pushup position, with your weight supported by your hands and toes. Flexing the knee and hip, bring one leg towards the corresponding arm. Explosively reverse the positions of your legs, extending the bent leg until the leg is straight and supported by the toe, and bringing the other foot up with the hip and knee flexed. Repeat in an alternating fashion.

Tap UPS

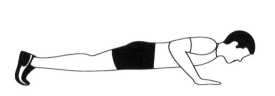 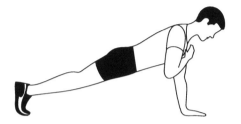

Begin in a pushup/plank position with your hands slightly wider than shoulder-width apart. Bend your elbows to lower your body to the floor just like a normal pushup. Pause, press back up to the starting position then tap one shoulder with the opposite side's hand. Repeat tapping the opposite shoulder.

★ TOP TIP ★

Work as hard as you can in each 30 sec burst. This is high intensity training so make you work your body as hard as you can while maintaining correct form for each exercise.

HIIT WORKOUT FOUR

- Exercise 1: **PRESS UPS** 20 secs | 10 secs rest
- Exercise 2: **SQUAT LUNGE** 20 secs | 10 secs rest
- Exercise 3: **STANDING STRAIGHT LEG BICYCLE** 20 secs | 10 secs rest
- Exercise 4: **TUCK JUMPS** 20 secs | 10 secs rest
- Exercise 5: **STANDING MOUNTAIN CLIMBERS** 20 secs | 10 secs rest
- Exercise 6: **BURPEES** 20 secs | 10 sec rest
- Exercise 6: **SCISSOR JUMPS** 20 secs | 2 minute rest

Repeat for 2 more sets

Perform each exercise as many times as possible within 30 seconds or hold for the desired length of time depending on the drill. Rest for 10 seconds then perform the next exercise again for 30 secs with a 10 sec rest in between exercises. Repeat until all 6 exercises have been completed.

Rest for 2 minutes then repeat the whole set two more times with a 2 minute rest in between.

Press UPS

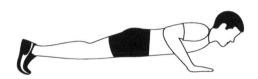

Begin in a high plank position with your hands shoulder-width apart. Lower your body ensuring you keep it aligned and look ahead to avoid strain in the neck. When your chest brushes the floor push back up. If you find this move difficult, start with your knees on the floor lowering only your upper torso.

Squat LUNGE

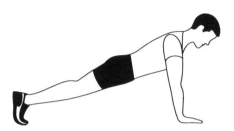

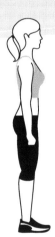

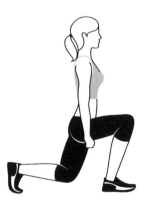

Stand upright with feet hip-width apart and arms at your sides. Take a controlled step forward with your right leg, keeping balance so that both knees are at 90 degree angles. Make sure your hips are low and back is straight. Push back with your right leg to the starting position. Repeat on left leg.

Standing Straight Leg BICYCLE

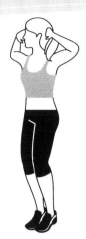
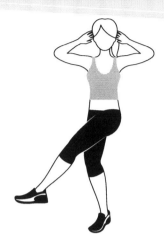

Begin by standing tall, hands touching the sides of your head but not clasped, feet shoulder-width apart. Opening your elbows wide, bring your right elbow down while simultaneously raising your left knee till they meet. Return to the starting position then repeat with left elbow to right knee. Opposite elbows go to opposite knees.

Tuck JUMP

Begin in a standing position with knees slightly bent and arms at your sides. Bend your knees and lower your body quickly into a squat position, then explosively jump upwards bringing your knees up towards your chest.

Standing MOUNTAIN CLIMBER

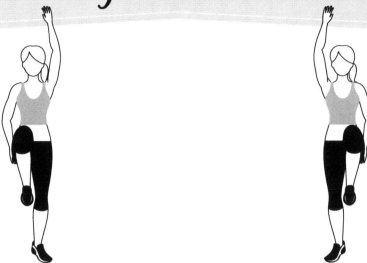

Begin by standing with feet shoulder-width apart and arms by your side. Bring your left knee up to waist level while extending your right arm to the sky. Return to the starting position then repeat this time raising your right knee and left arm. Keep alternating sides in a climbing motion.

Burpees

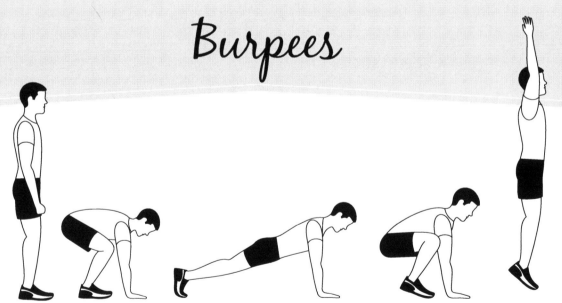

Lie on your back and extend your arms out to the side. Raise your knees and feet so they create a 90-degree angle. Contract your abdominals and exhale as you lift your hips off the floor. Your knees will move toward your head. Try to keep your knees at a right angle. Inhale and slowly lower.

Scissor JUMPS

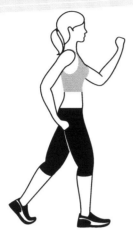 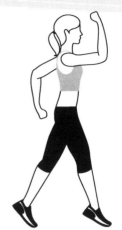

Begin by standing with right foot approx. 2 feet in front of left. Right arm should be extended behind you and left arm in front of you with elbows bent as if in a running position. Quickly jump up while switching arm and leg positions while in the air, landing with left foot in front of right foot and right arm in front of your body, left arm behind you. Continue alternating arms and legs while jumping.

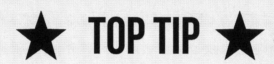

★ TOP TIP ★

Keep your core tight! By keeping your abdominal area firm, not only are you working the ab muscles but also keeping a strong mid-section which is vital for balance and control.

Straight Leg Calf STRETCH

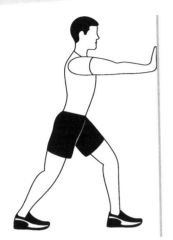 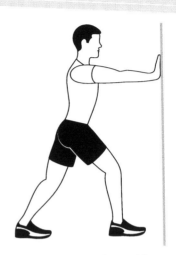

Place both hands on a wall with arms extended. Lean against the wall with right leg bent forward and left leg extended behind with knee straight and feet positioned directly forward. Push rear heal to floor and move hips slightly forward holding the stretch for 10 secs. Repeat with opposite leg.

Shoulder STRETCH

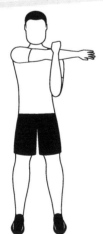 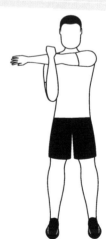

The right arm is placed over the left shoulder. Position the wrist on your left arm to the elbow of your right arm gently pushing towards the shoulder. Swap shoulders.

Standing Quadricep STRETCH

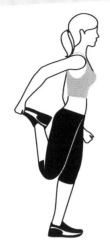 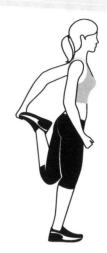

Begin by standing with your feet hip-width apart. Bend your right leg backwards grasping the right foot to bring your heel toward your buttocks. Hold for 5-10 secs then repeat for left leg. Use your opposite arm to balance if need be.

Lower Back STRETCH

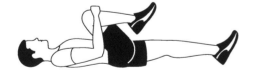 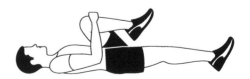

Begin by lying flat on your back with toes pointed upward. Slowly bend your right knee and pull your leg up to you chest, wrapping your arms around your thigh and hands clasped around the knee or shin. Gently pull the knee towards your chest and hold for 10 secs. Repeat on left leg.

Cat Cow STRETCH

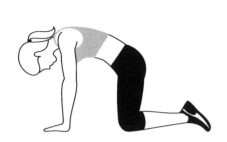 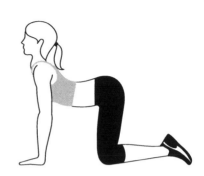

Begin with your hands and knees on the floor. Exhale while rounding your spine up towards the ceiling, pulling your belly button up towards your spine, and engaging your core. Inhale while arching your back and letting your tummy relax.

 CookNation

Other COOKNATION TITLES

If you enjoyed **The** *Skinny* **NUTRiBULLET Lean Body** *HIIT* **Plan** you may also be interested in other *Skinny* **NUTRiBULLET** titles in the CookNation series.

Visit **www.bellmackenzie.com** to browse the full catalogue.

Printed in Great Britain
by Amazon